Adult Dot to Dot Book of
Butterflies and Flowers

COLOR TEST PAGE

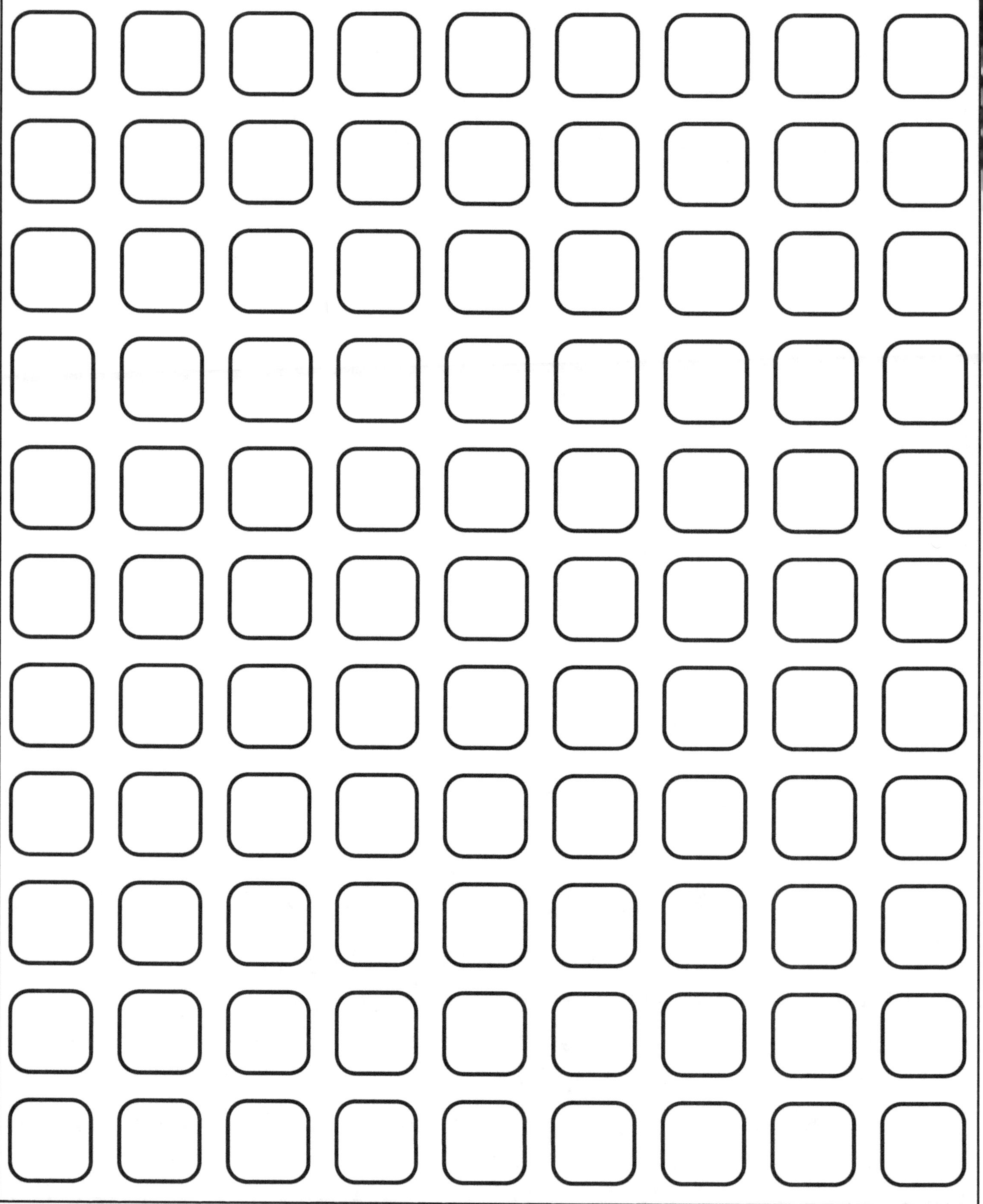

COLOR TEST PAGE

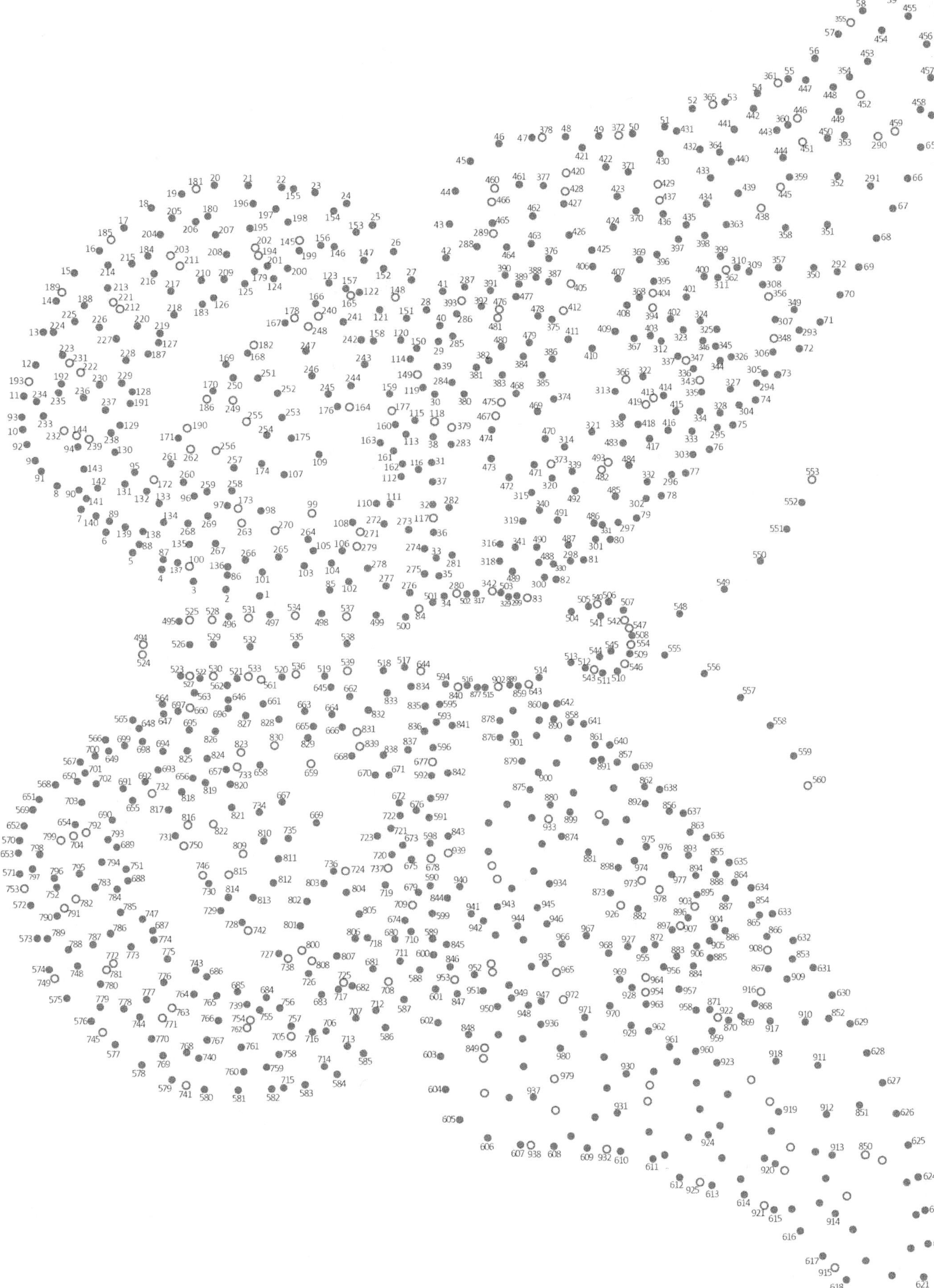

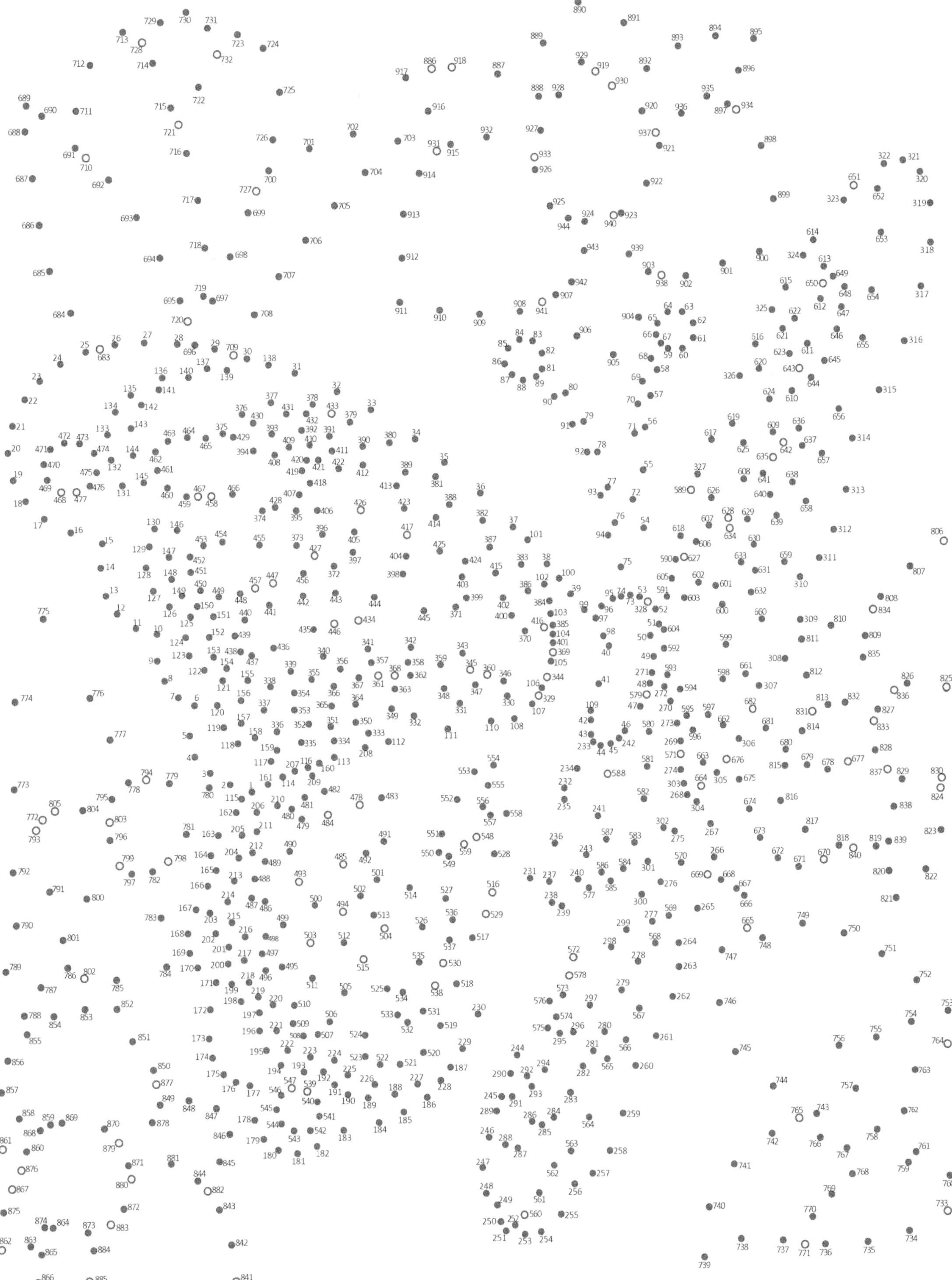

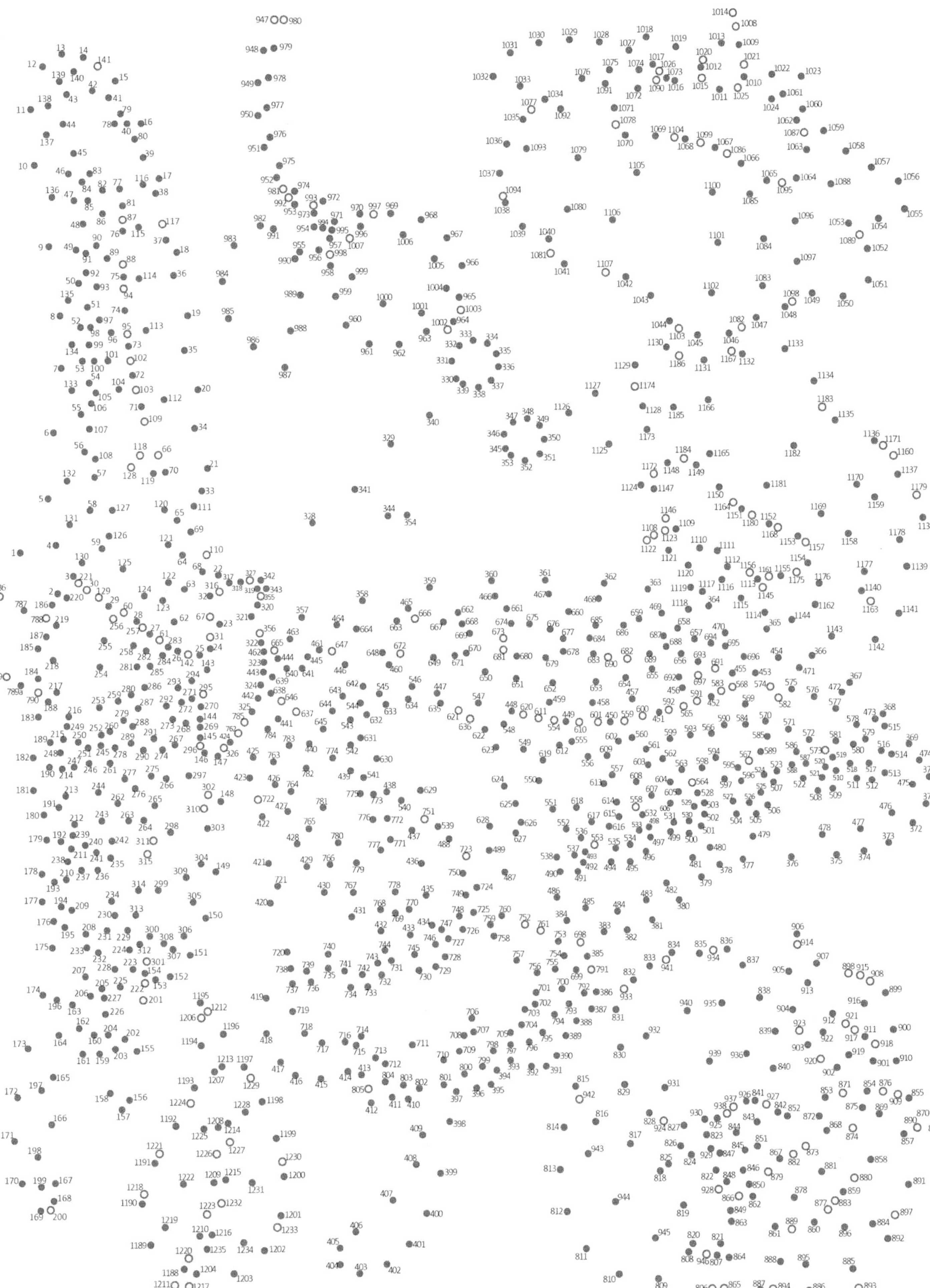

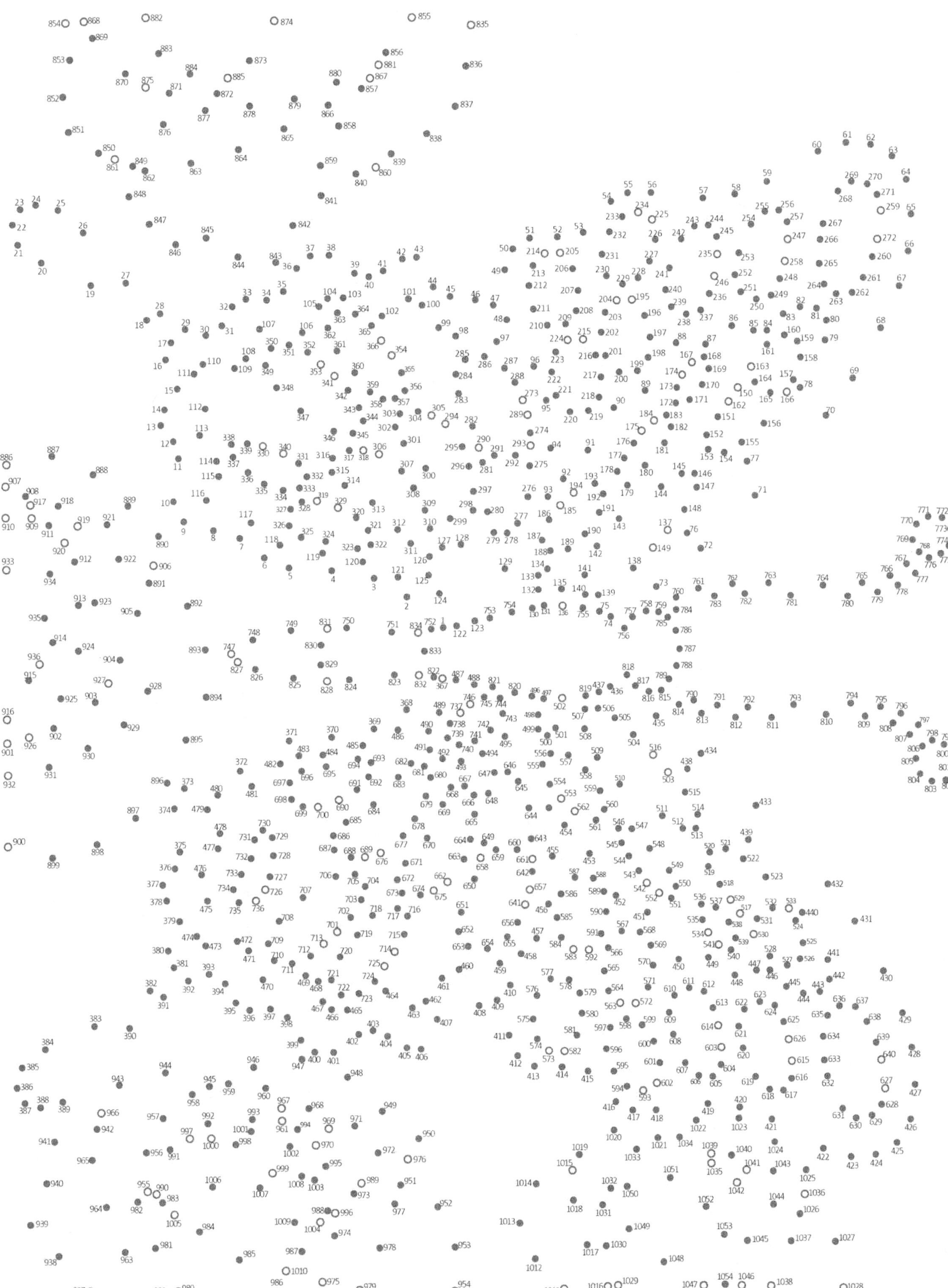

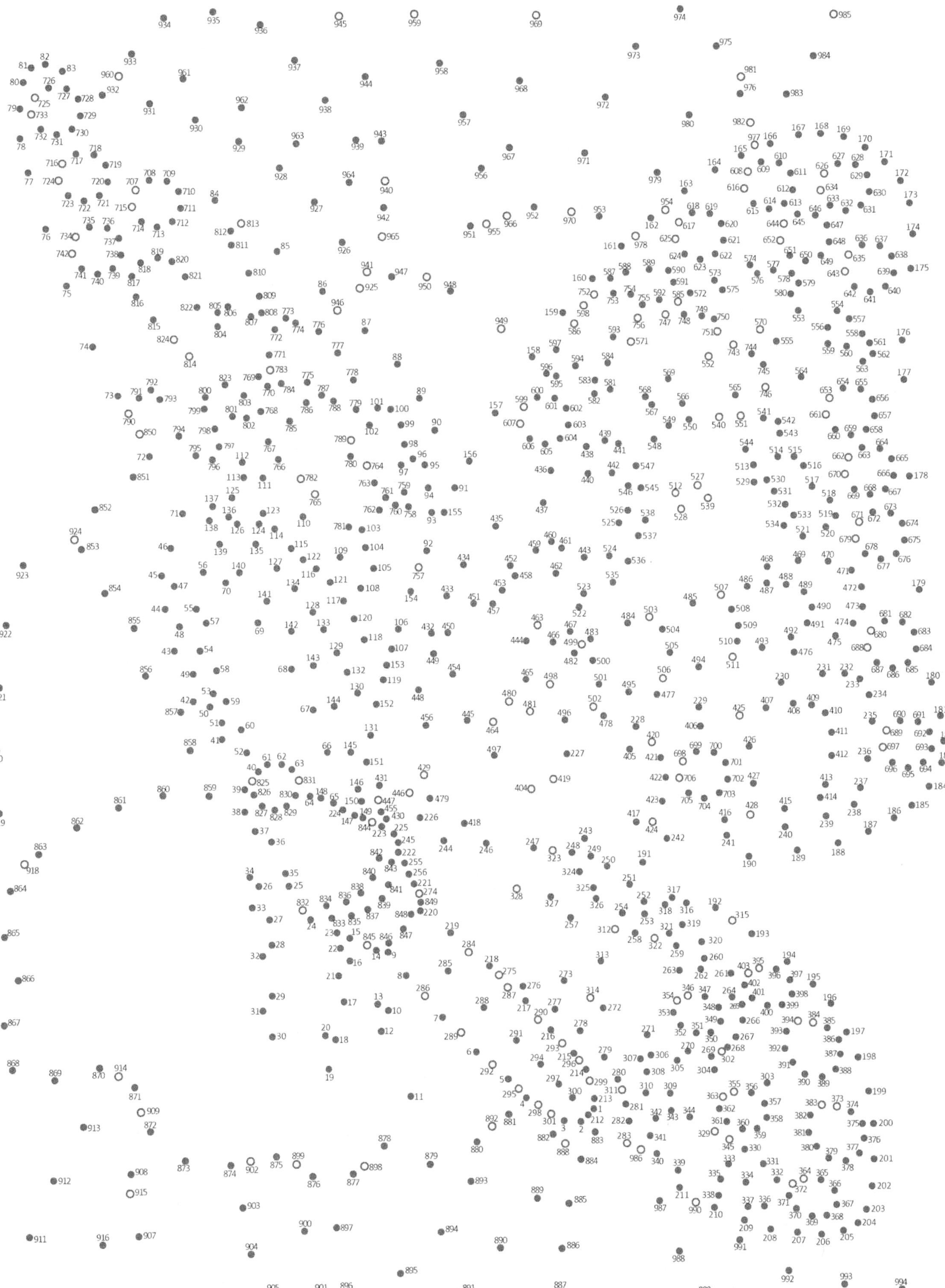

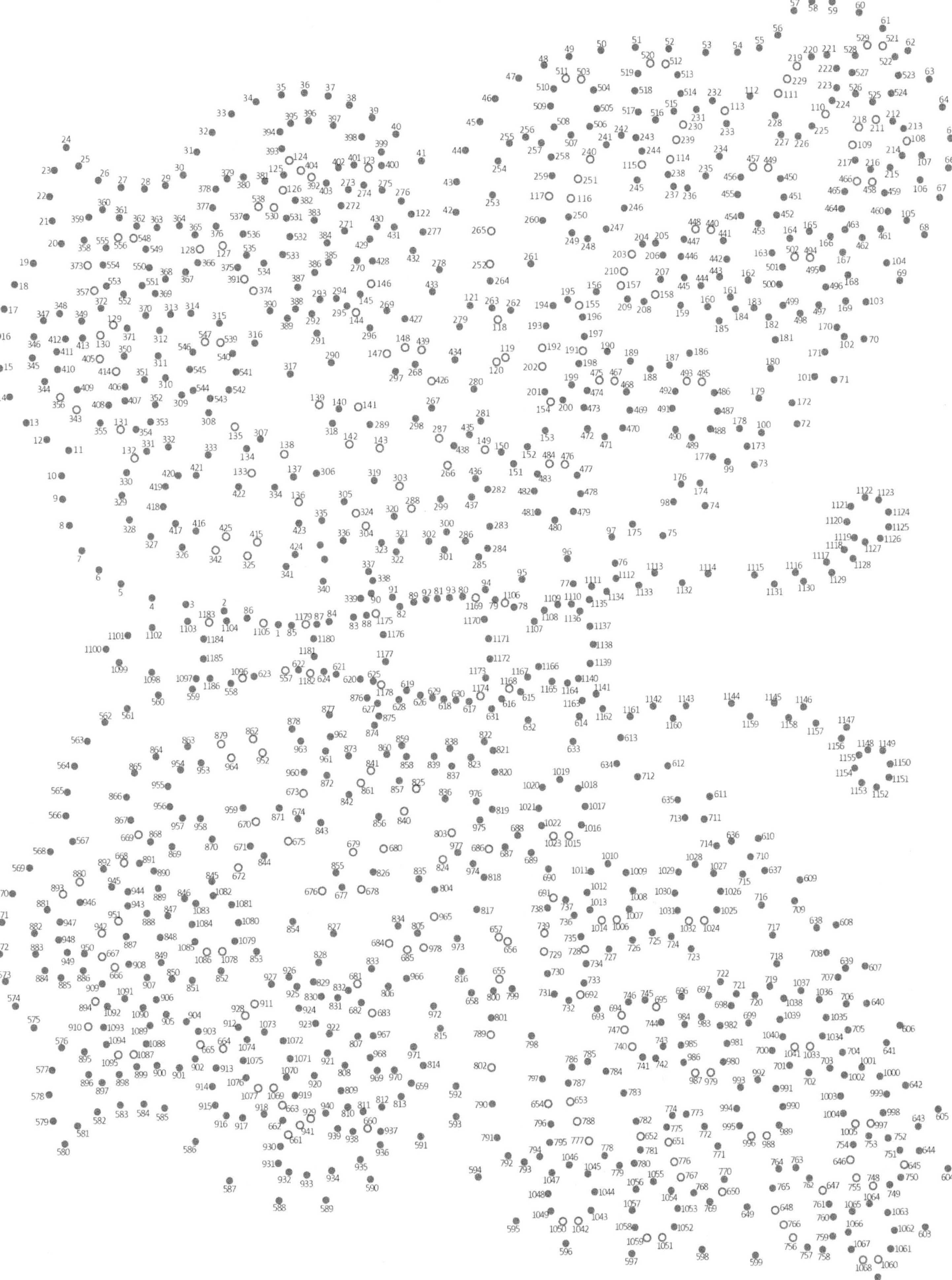

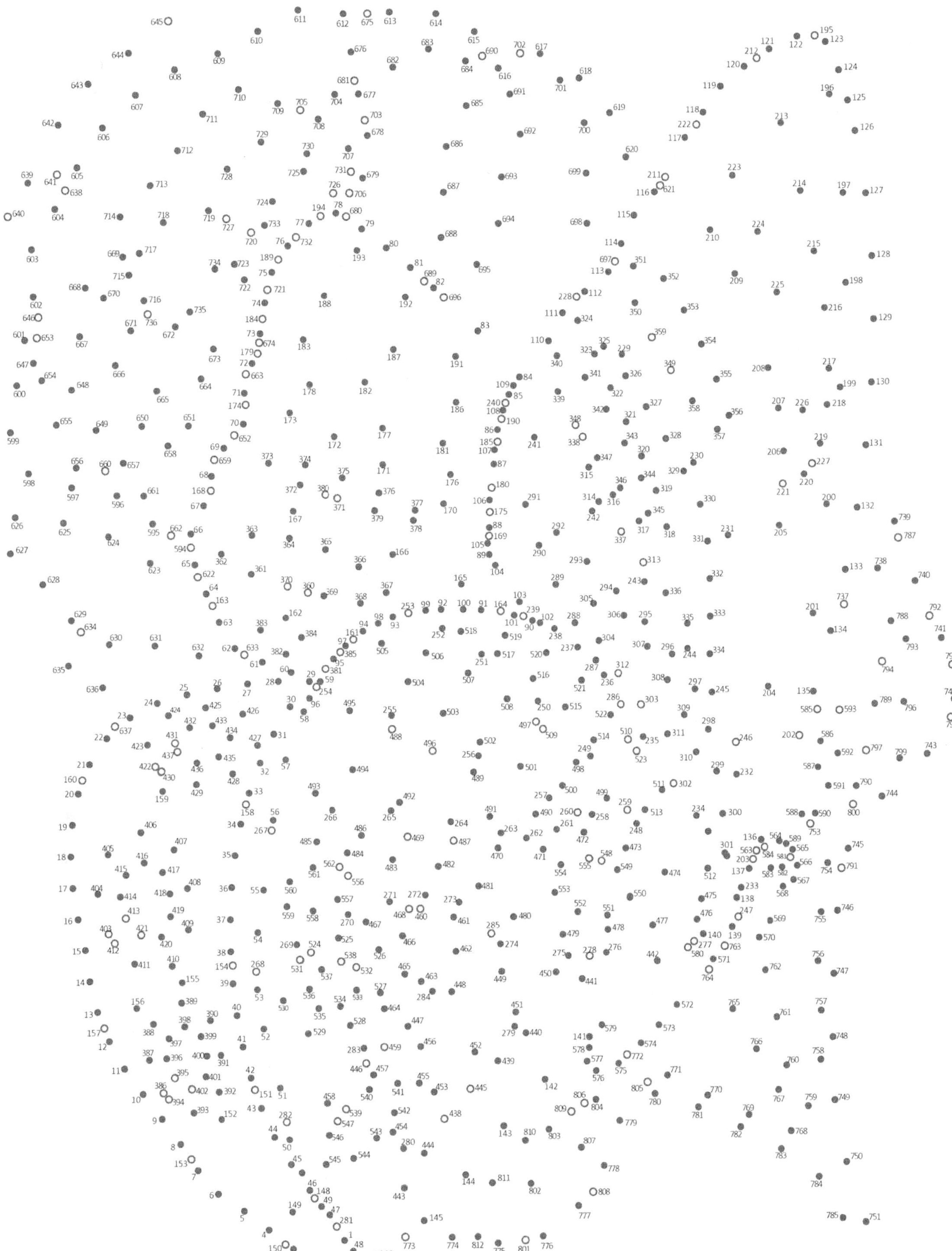

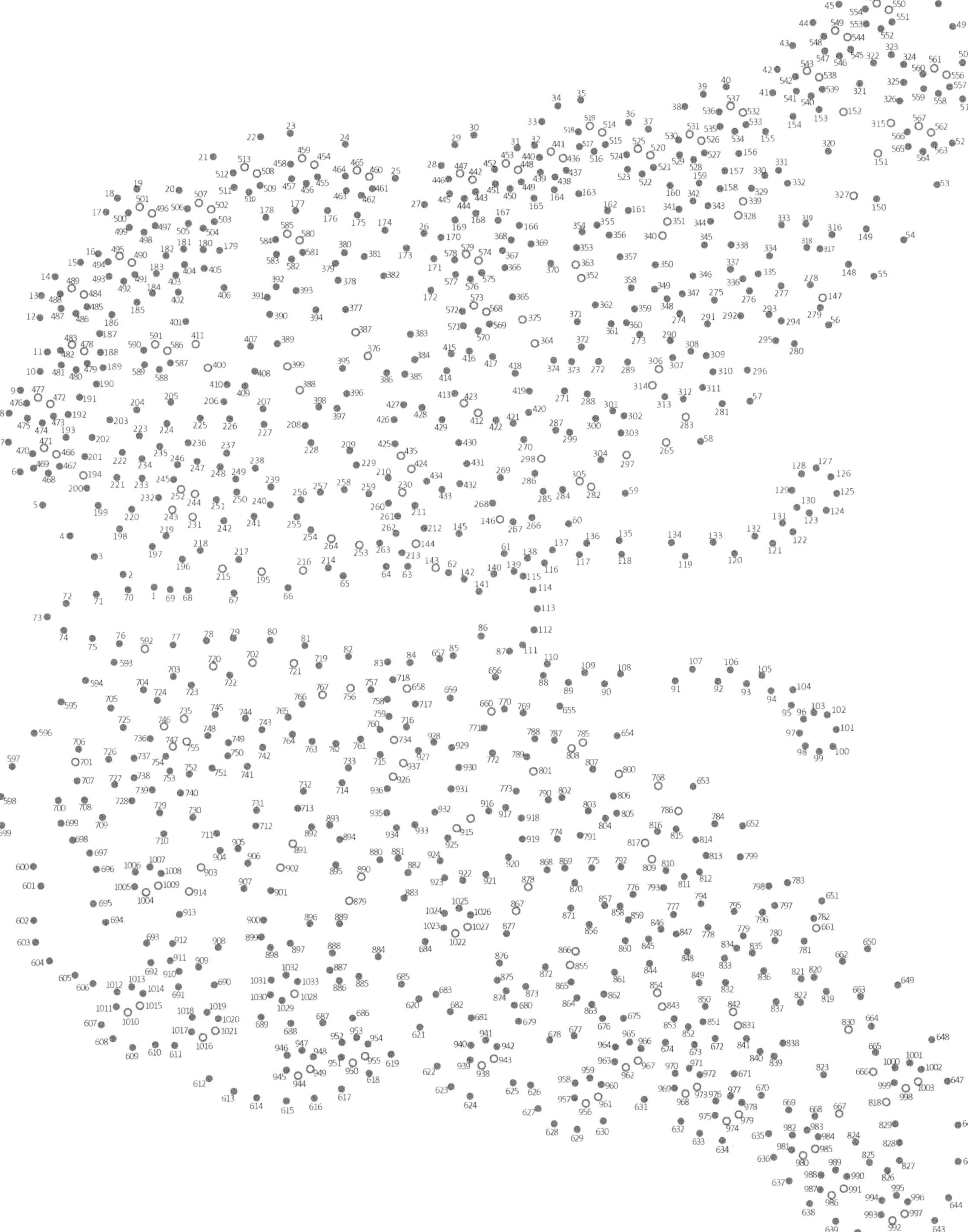

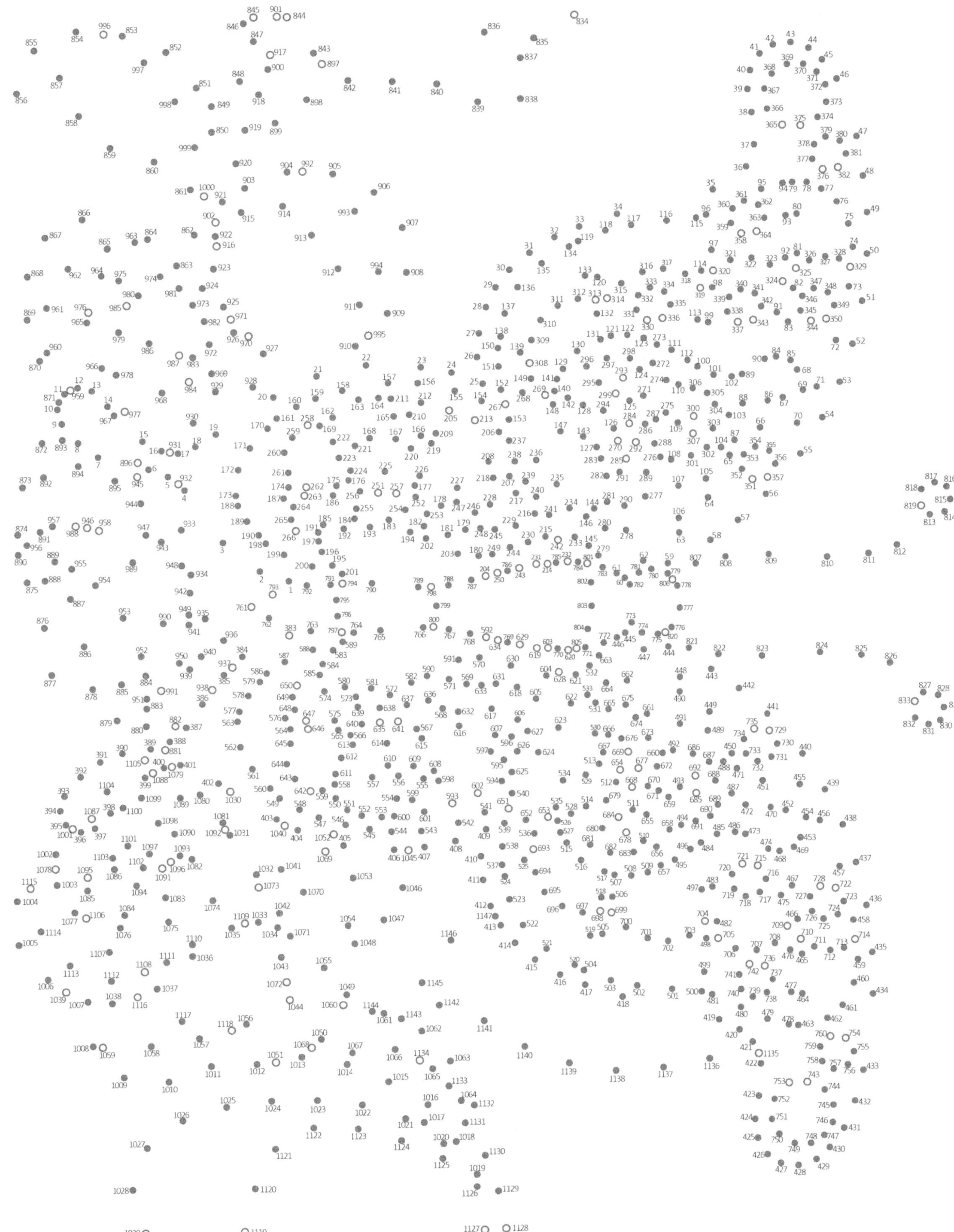

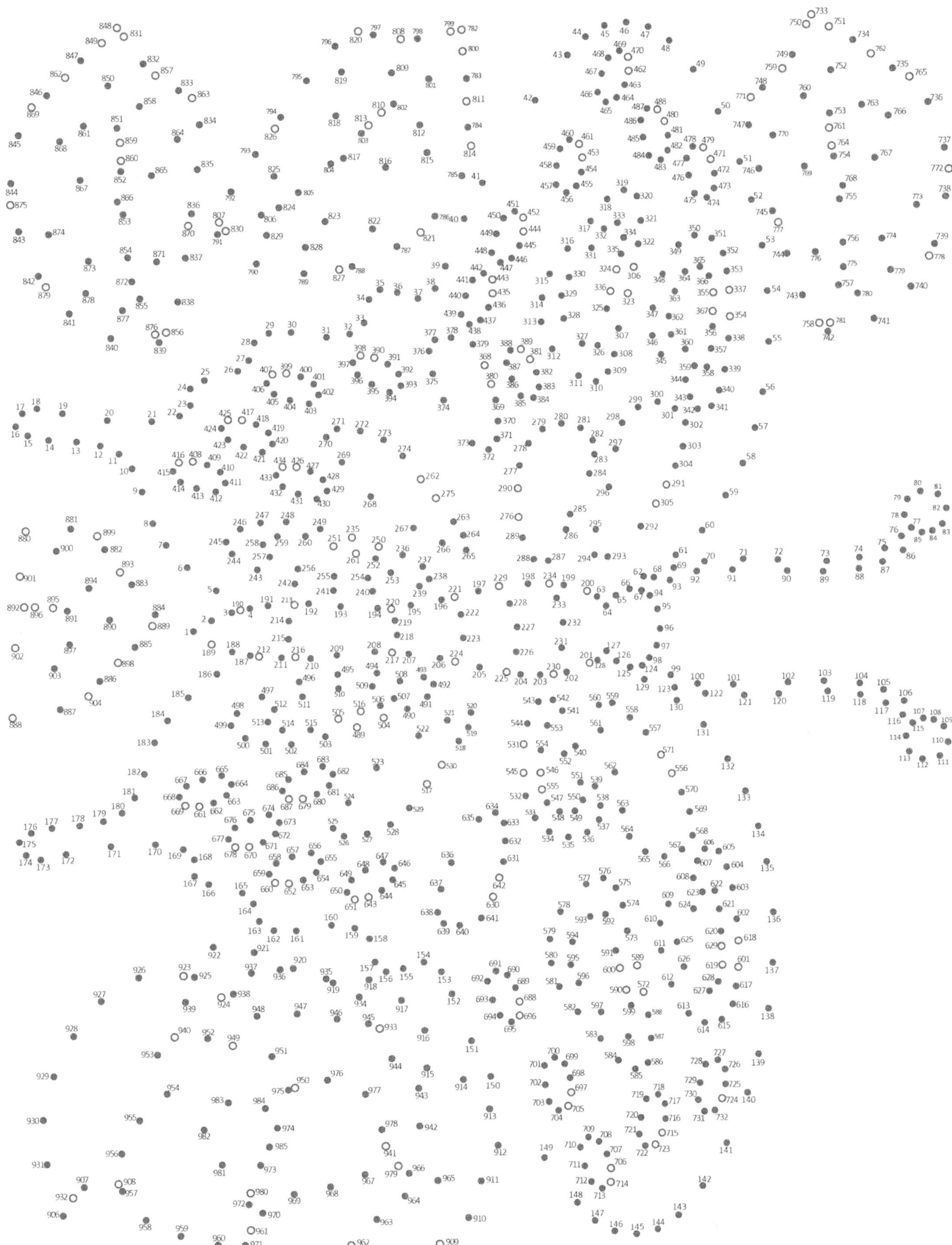

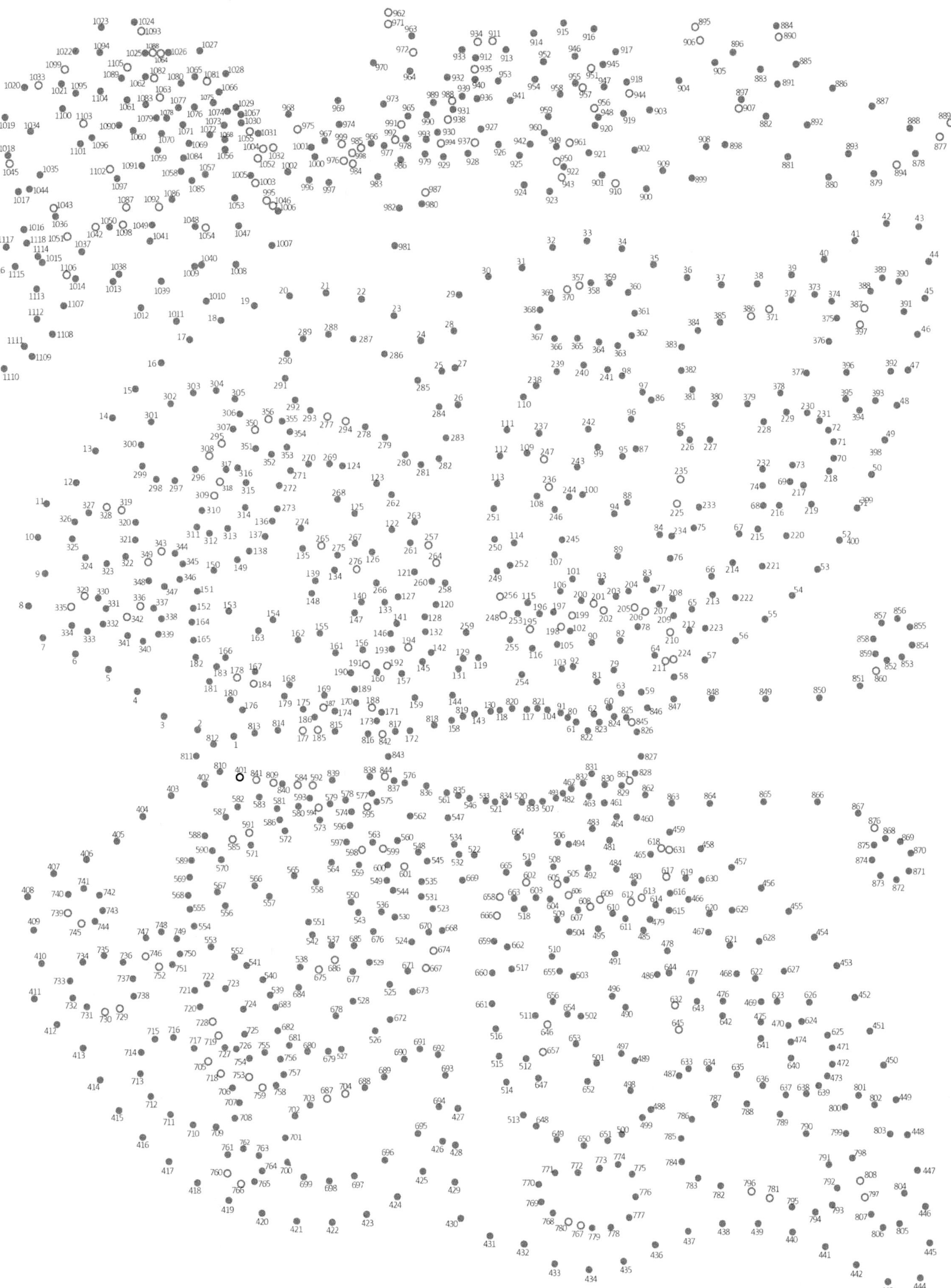

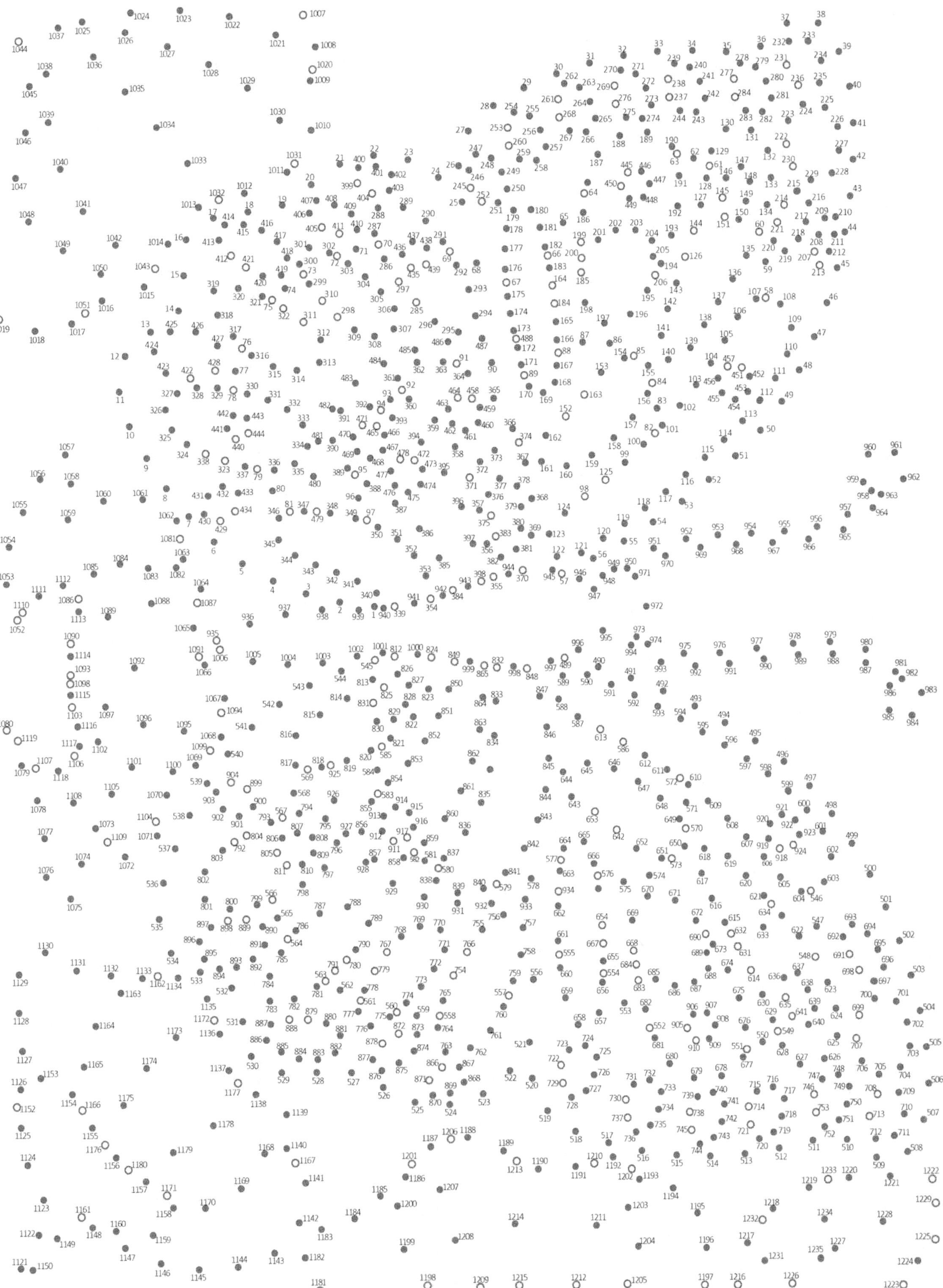

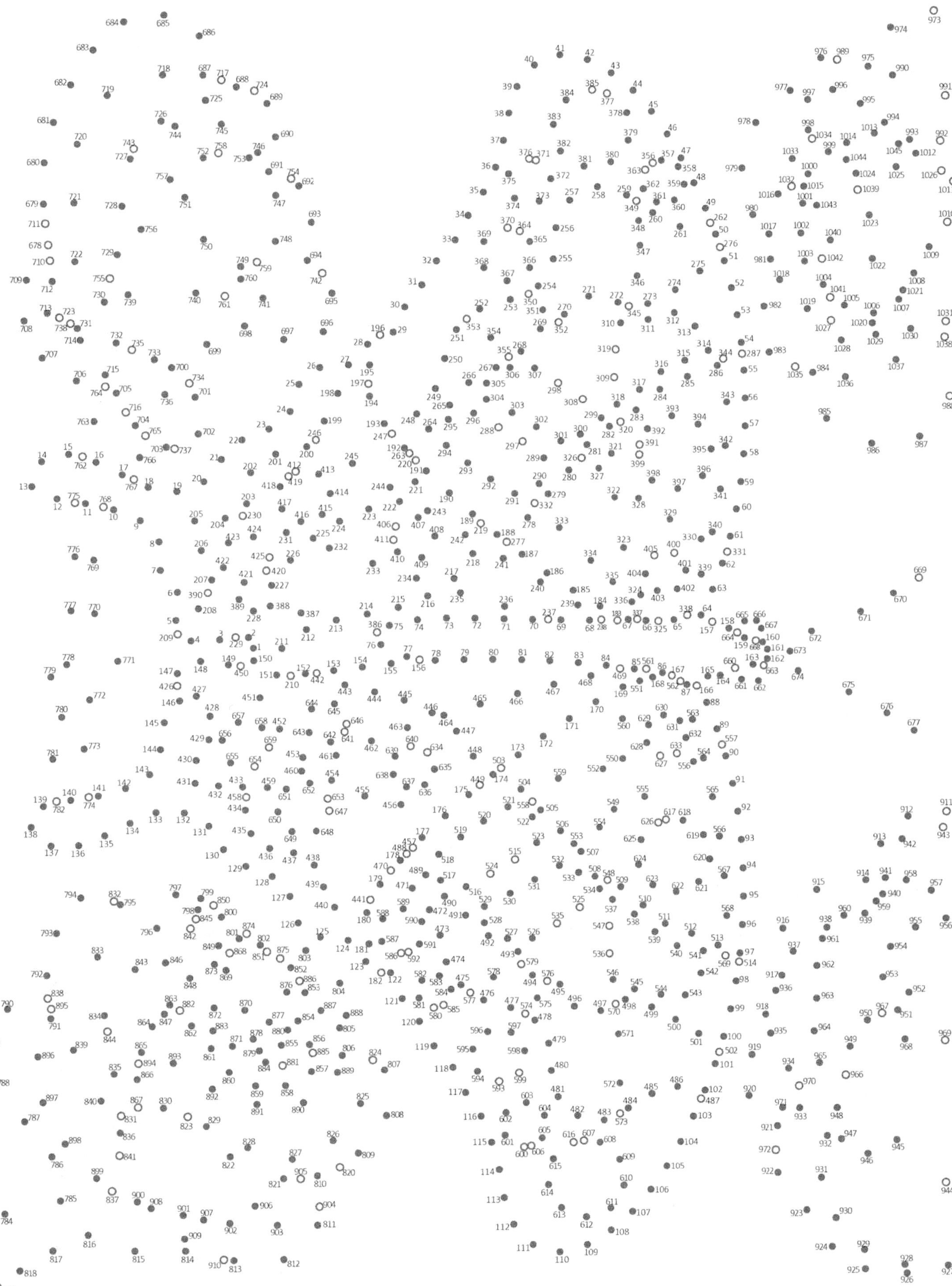

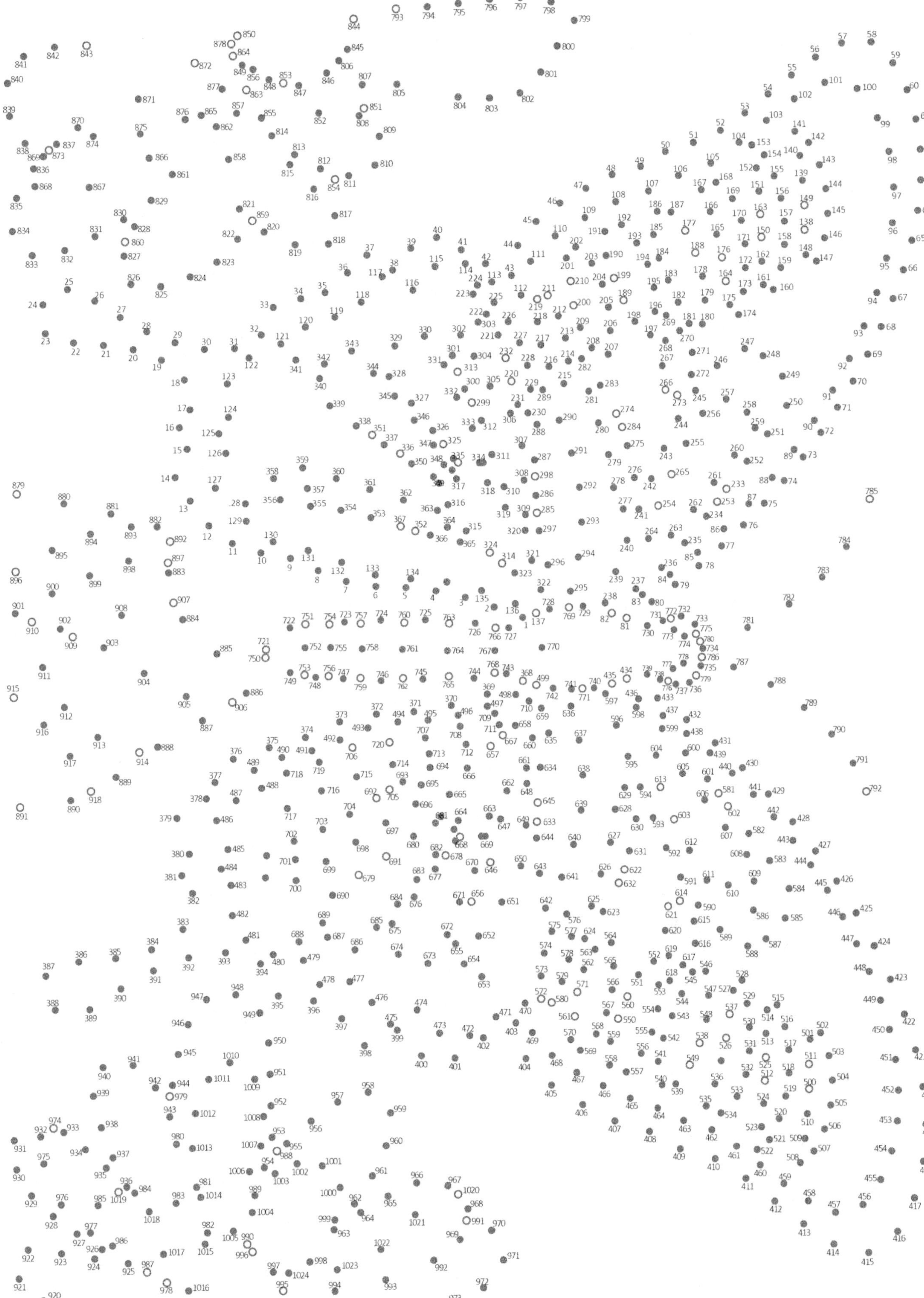

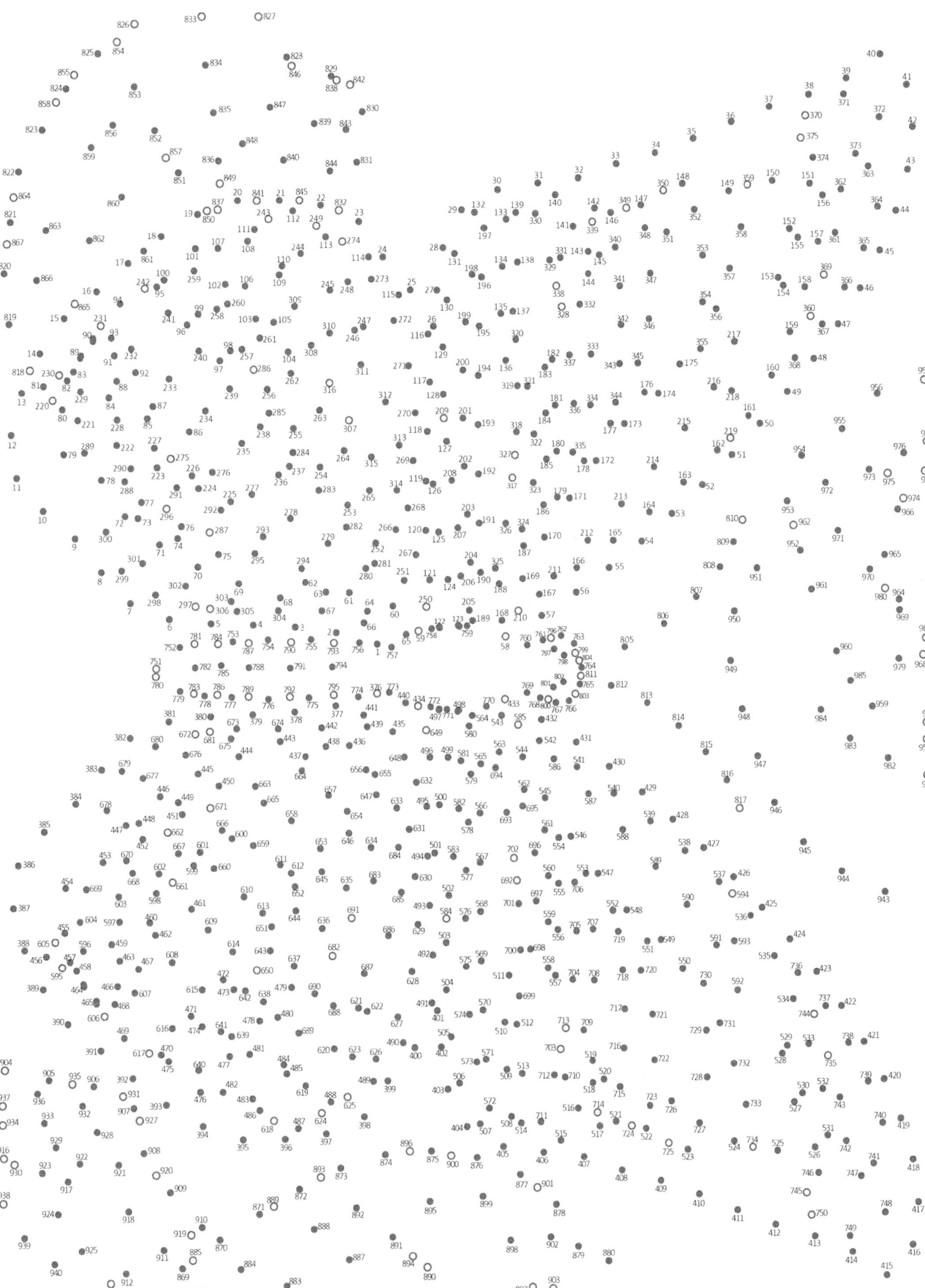

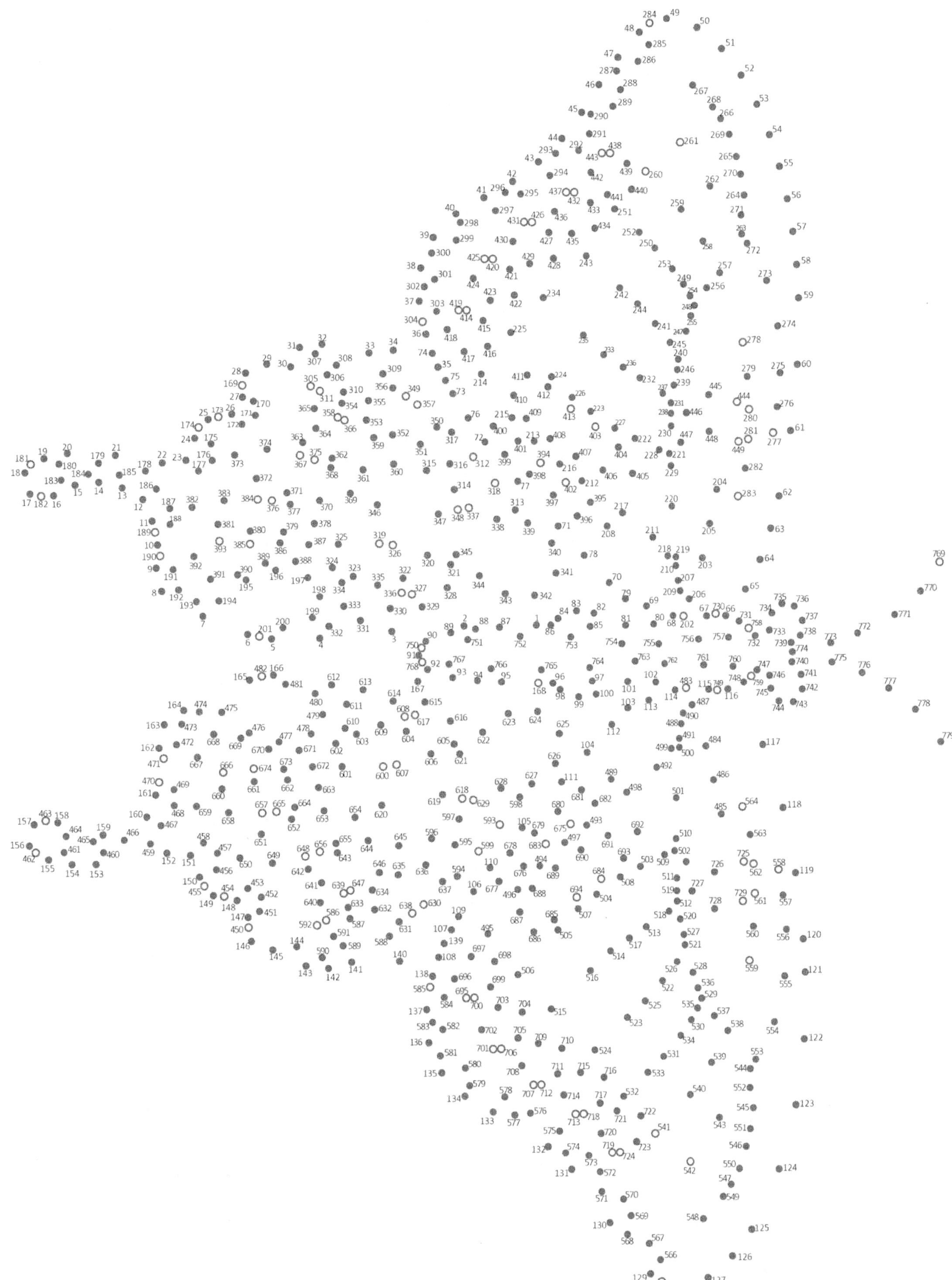

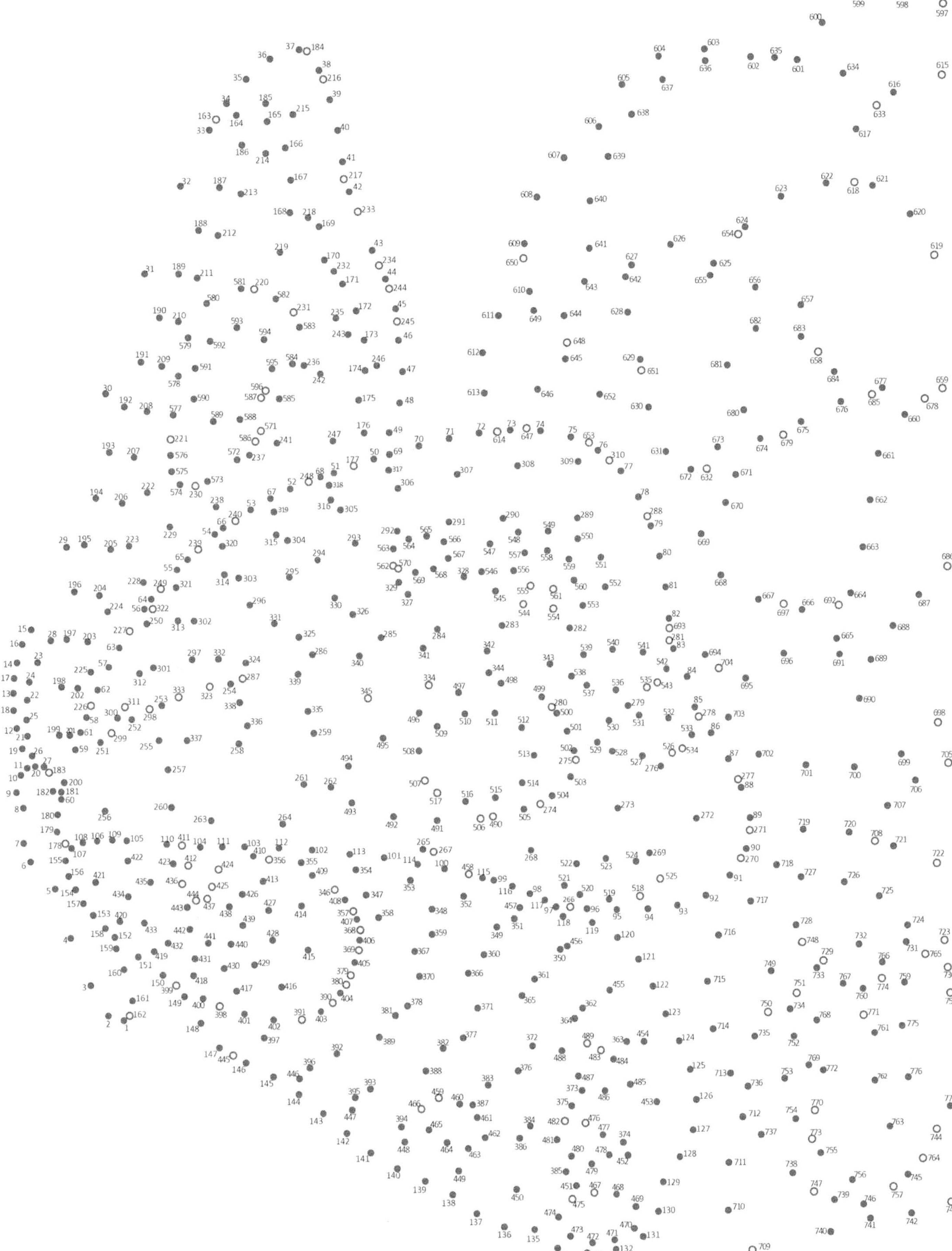

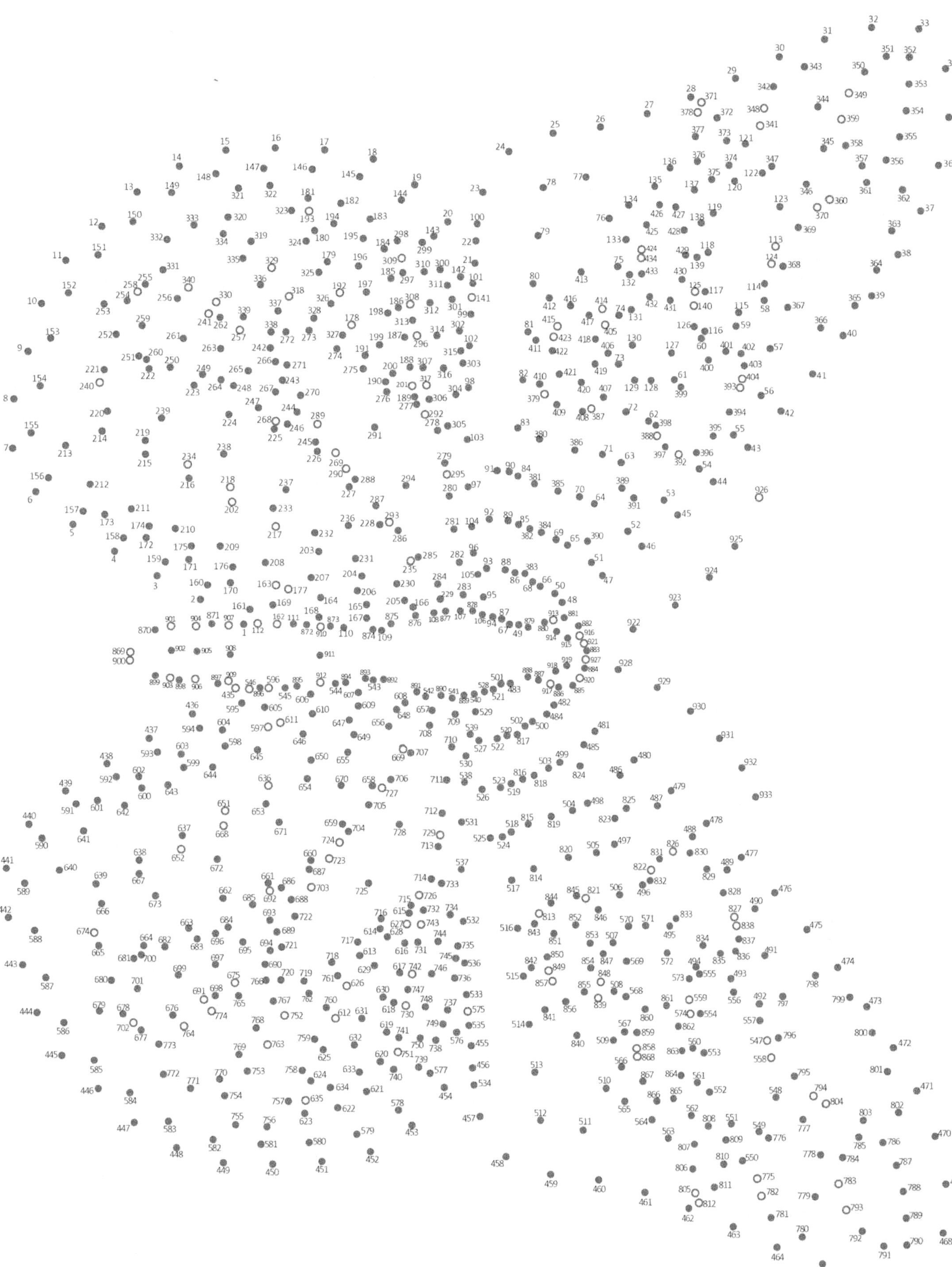

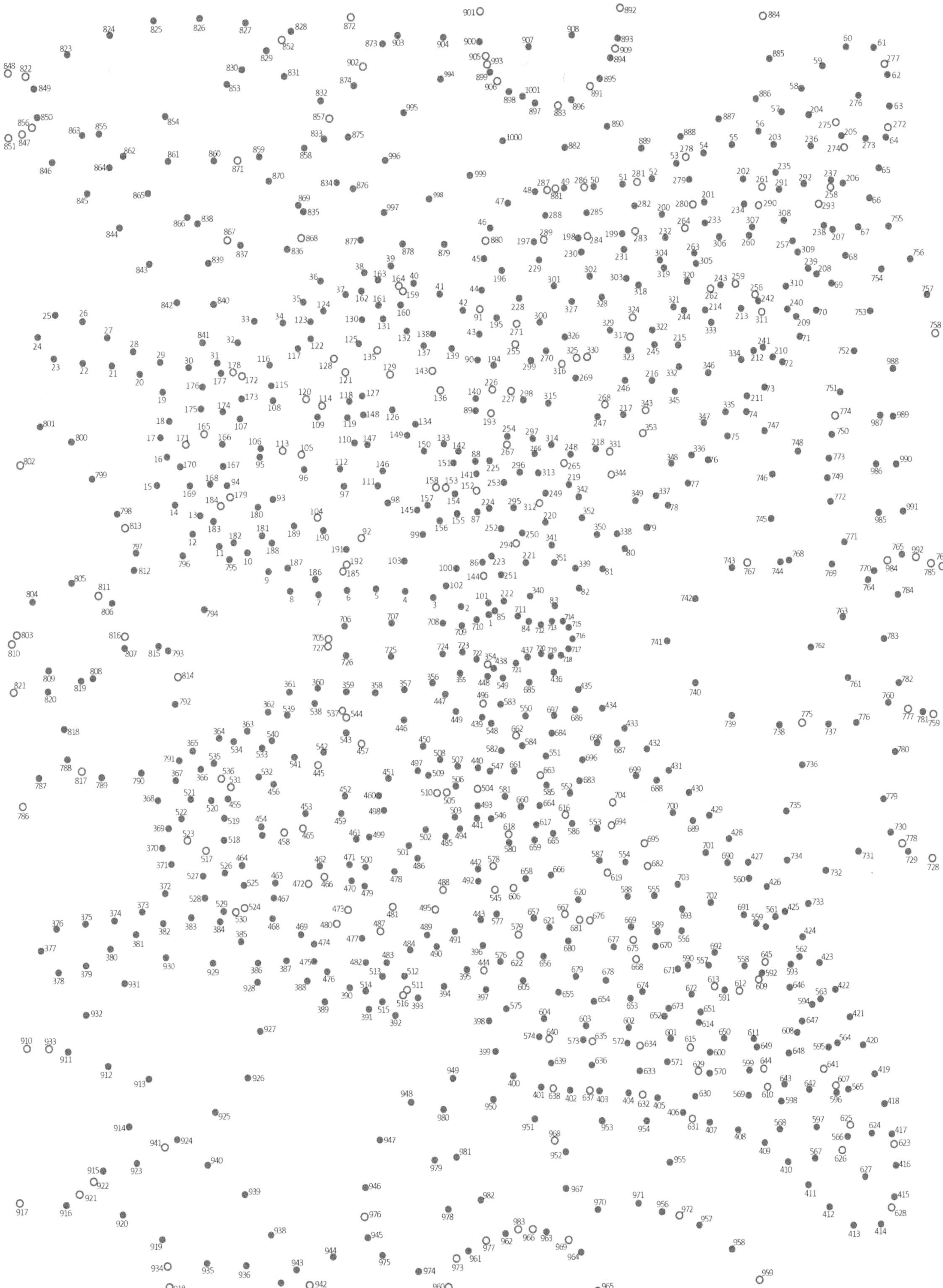

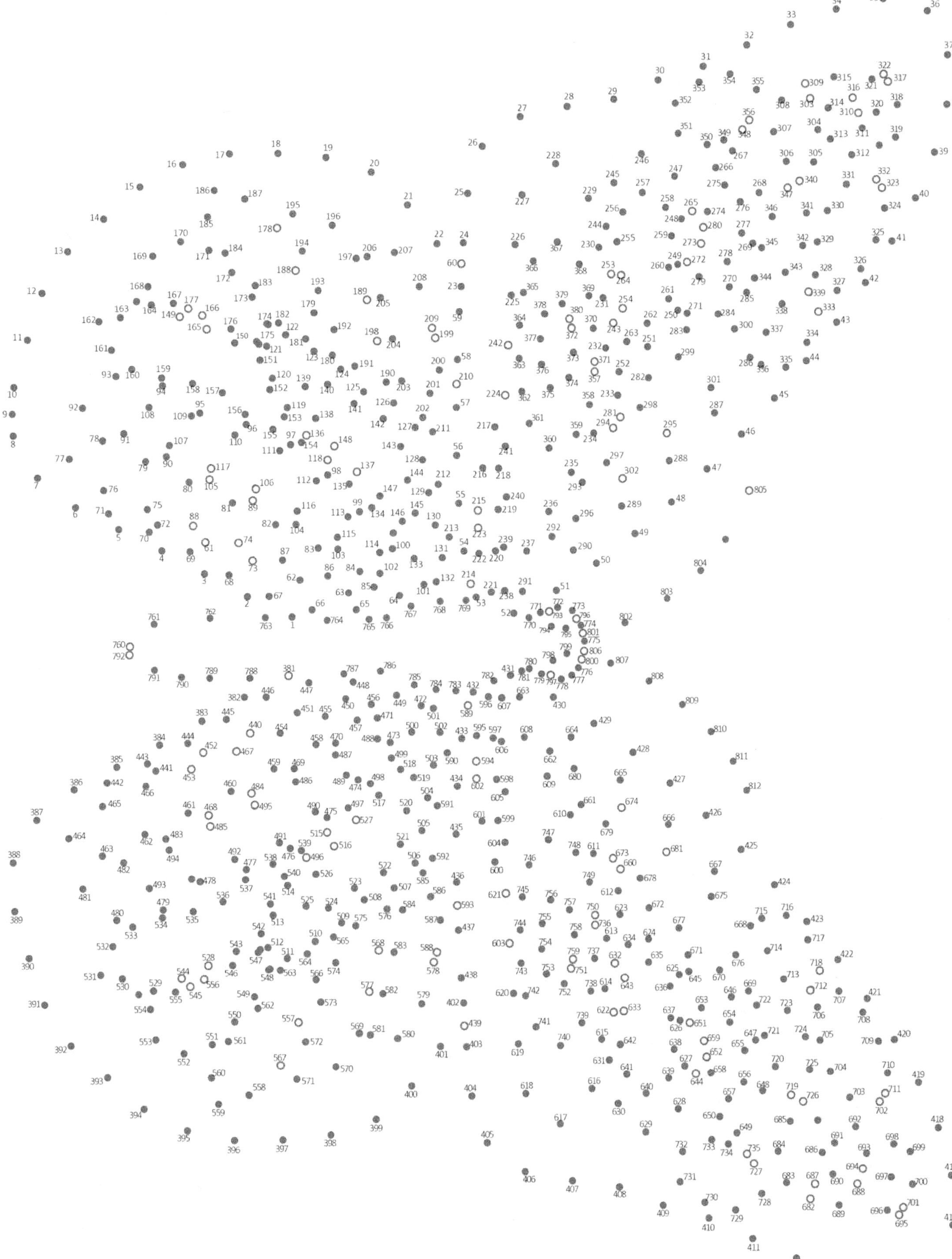

Thank you for supporting
ZenMaster Coloring Books

Your support means the world to us,
and we're thrilled to have you embark on this
creative journey with us.

Our small company strives to make a
BIG difference by helping those
who may be less fortunate.

This is why we proudly hire struggling
artists from around the world!

Our goal is to provide financial support to artists and
their families by enabling them to pursue their passions
and share their hard work and limitless talent with you!

Help support our hard working artists
by leaving a positive review on Amazon!

And follow us on Facebook for updates and
FREE COLORING PAGES!
https://www.facebook.com/zenmastercoloringbooks/

Check out more of our books at:
amazon.com/author/zenmastercoloringbooks

Free Bonus Page!
from:

Happy Summer
coloring book for adults

https://www.amazon.com/dp/1986950115

Also available in color by numbers!!
https://www.amazon.com/dp/1986983838

And a 5x8" Travel Size
https://www.amazon.com/dp/172614500X

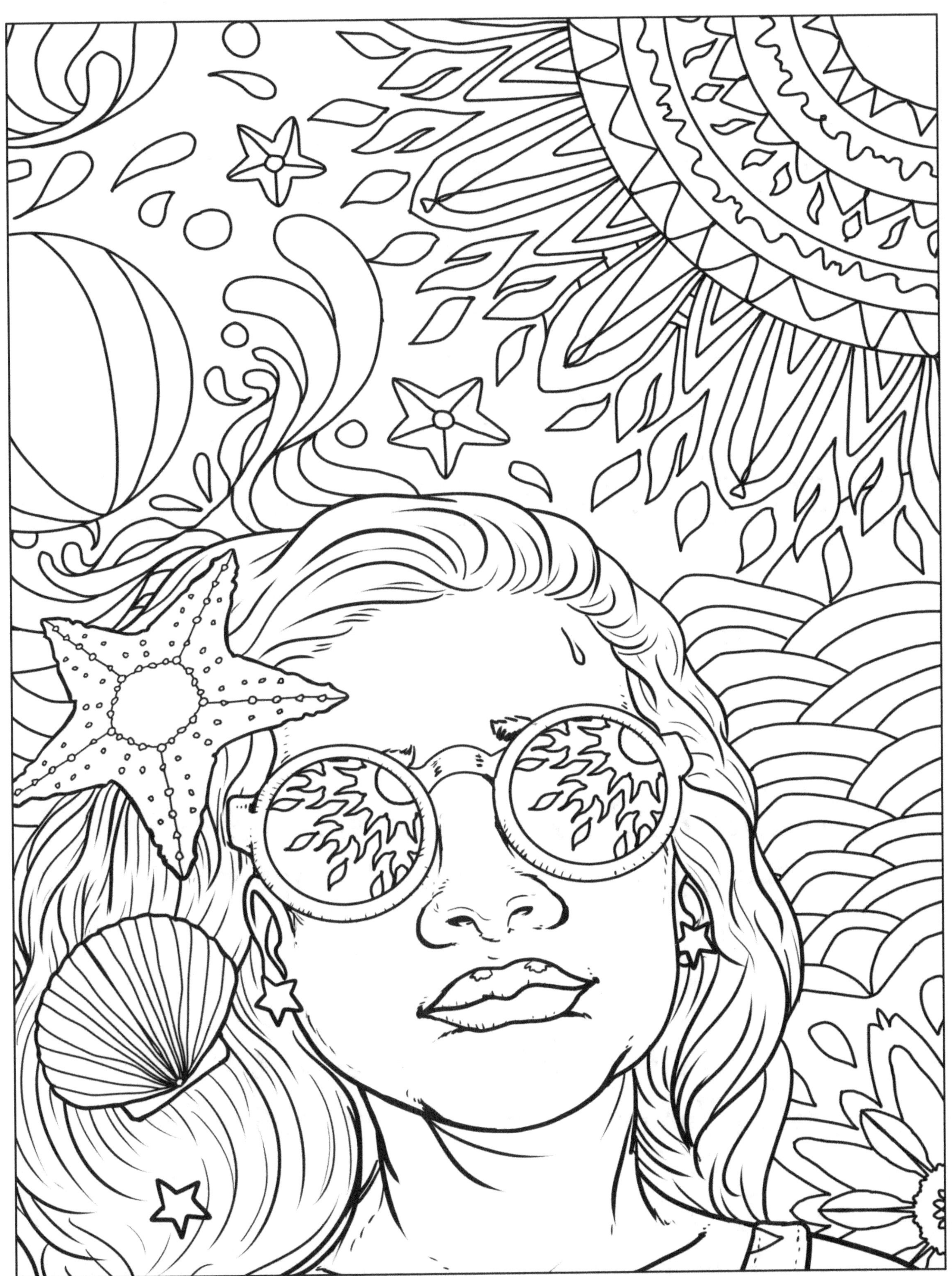

Free Bonus Page!
from:

Adult Coloring Book of
Island Dreams Vacation

https://www.amazon.com/dp/1976291267

Also available in color by numbers!!
https://www.amazon.com/dp/1976507707

And 5x8" Travel Size
https://www.amazon.com/dp/1796516090

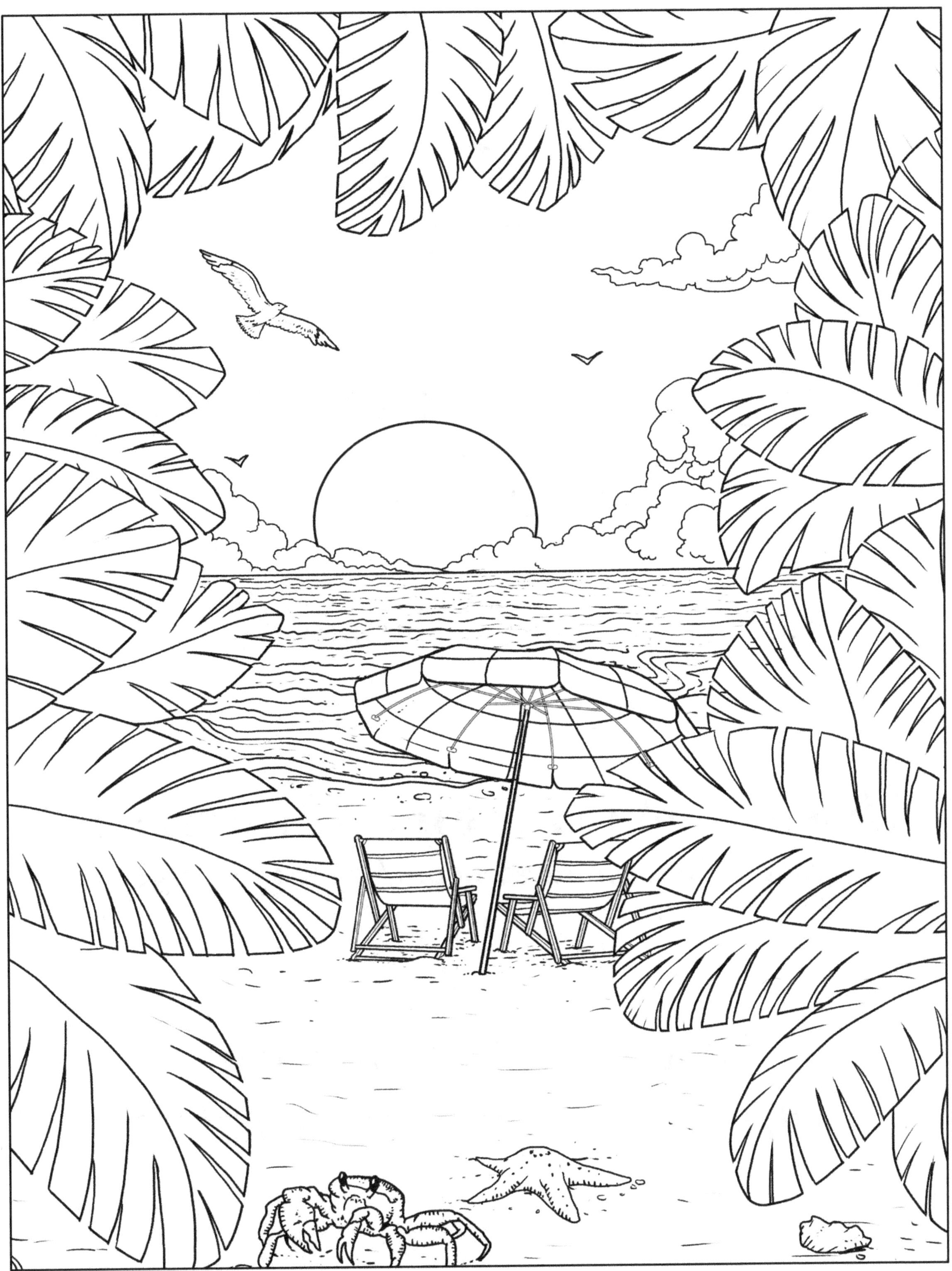

Free Bonus Page!
from:

Large Print Adult Coloring Book of
Dachshunds

https://www.amazon.com/dp/1977508456

Also available in color by numbers!!
https://www.amazon.com/dp/1977842658

And 5x8" Travel Size
https://www.amazon.com/dp/1977576079

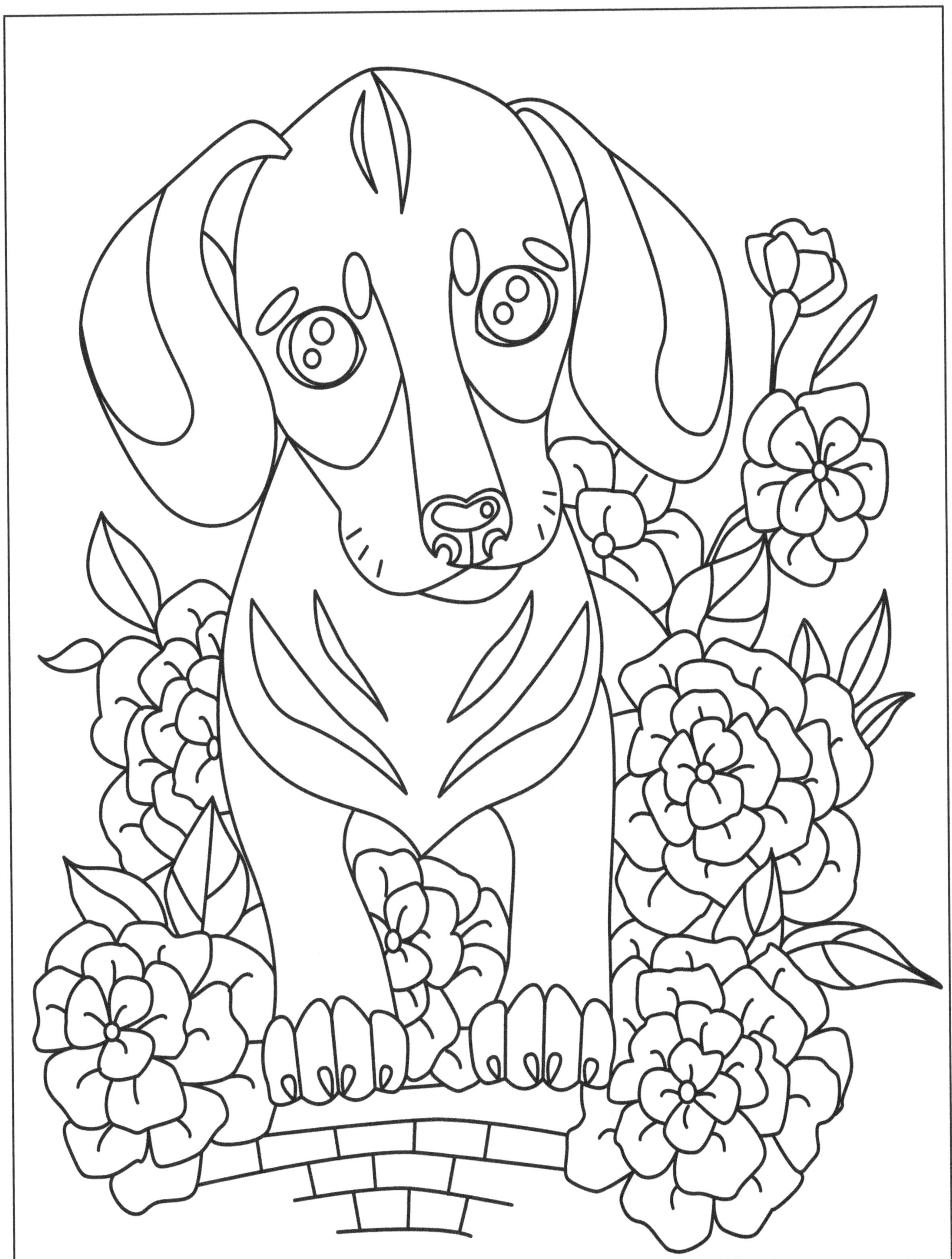